This book is dedicated to my cherished partner Agi ... who never dumped me even when I looked hideous ☺

Richard James Clapham P.hD. Bioinspired Robotics
© 2016 copyright

EYE CHALAZION TREATMENT: How to remove without surgery

The Methods I Used For Success!

2nd Edition

By Richard James Clapham

Disclaimer:

This book is not intended as a substitute for the medical advice of physicians. The reader should regularly consult a physician in matters relating to his/her health and particularly with respect to any symptoms that may require diagnosis or medical attention. Although the author and publisher have made every effort to ensure that the information in this book was correct at press time, the author and publisher do not assume and hereby disclaim any liability to any party for any loss, damage, or disruption caused by errors or omissions, whether such errors or omissions result from negligence, accident, or any other cause. The information provided in this book is designed to provide helpful information on the subjects discussed. This book is not meant to be used, nor should it be used, to diagnose or treat any medical condition. For diagnosis or treatment of any medical problem, consult your own physician. The publisher and author are not responsible for any specific health or allergy needs that may require medical supervision and are not liable for any damages or negative consequences from any treatment, action, application or preparation, to any person reading or following the information in this book. References are provided for informational purposes only and do not constitute endorsement of any websites or other sources. Readers should be aware that the websites listed in this book may change.

ABSTRACT

This book is the result of my successful attempt to conquer my large swollen eye chalazion which I had for months.

After understanding the causes of a chalazion and styes, I tested various methods to remove the lump from my eye, resulting in the chalazion swelling completely disappearing from draining away, by using a smooth and soft approach where no cutting or piecing the skin was required.

The widely spread technique described online of applying warm compresses does not typically work. It really didn't work for me. I didn't want to undergo surgery and there are some really gruesome videos about showing a cutting and removal approach which made me even more determined to find a successful solution.

My focus was to read and understand as much as possible, identify what I had and its causes. After this intensive investigation I began to realise how I could possibly drain the chalazion carefully. My methods thoroughly described in the following chapters almost guarantee to reduce your swelling and hopefully avoid the last resort of taking the lump out whole.

This book is short and concise. I didn't want to pad or waffle on we just want to start getting that lump disappearing.

CONTENTS

INTRODUCTION

This section briefly identifies the different types of eye swellings which can occur and the recommended methods which are widely known to treat them. For detailed information please uses the references provided in Section 5. The information in this Section is easily found on the internet and can be skipped if you are sure of your condition. Firstly we must understand which type of blockage you have. The two prominent types are listed below:

Stye:

A stye can be described as an infection that causes a tender red sore lump located near the outer edge of the eyelid usually caused by an infected eyelash follicle. They look similar to a pimple or spot. Most styes swell for typically three days and then burst open and drain and are healed within a week. An internal stye is called a hordeolum which is caused by an infection in an oil gland. If a hordeolum is unable to drain it will become a chalazion [5, 6, 9].

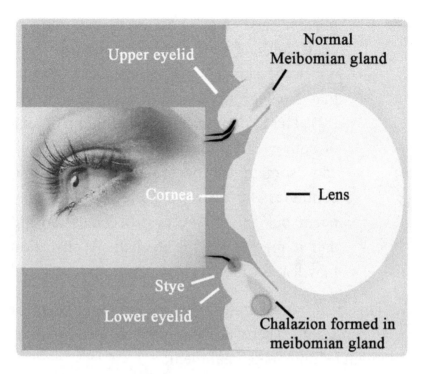

Fig 1: Showing the location of a stye, the meibomian gland and a chalazion.

*© Please reference this book and author if you wish to use this image.

Chalazion (Meibomian cyst):

A chalazion usually develops in a location further from the edge of the eyelid than a stye, as a chalazion forms when an oil gland in the eyelid becomes blocked. They may look like a stye but usually grow to be larger in size and may not even be sore. A chalazion can be described as a firm lump under the skin (A cyst is a cluster of cells that have grouped together to form a sac [8]). The Symptoms are a small lump on one or both eyelids, where mild pain or irritation can sometimes occur. If the swelling continues to grow distorted vision may occur but only if the cyst becomes too big and it presses on the eyeball. A chalazion may last for months [1, 2, 3, 4, 7].

This book concentrates on the condition known as a chalazion. There are three prominent methods given by doctors to heal them:

Warm compresses:
Treatment of the chalazion can be aided by applying warm compress to the affected location for approximately fifteen to twenty minutes four times per day. A technique used to soften the inflammation [12, 13, 14].

Antibiotics:
Antibiotics may be prescribed to reduce the inflammation in the eyelid. Please note the negative effects of antibiotic consumption

on the body should always be understood, such as allergic reactions [13, 14].

Surgery:
A surgical procedure called 'incision and curettage' will be typically undertaken if the inflammation does not show any signs of disappearing, in which the cyst is removed by cutting the inside of the eyelid. Smaller swellings may be first injected with a corticosteroid. If the lump continues to enlarge or does not stop growing within a few months after the injections it will usually need to be surgically removed using local anaesthesia, and some after treatment is recommend. The surgical procedure is nearly always successful. However, even after a positive surgery a chalazion can appear again. If this happens you may need another operation to remove it [1, 2, 10, 12, 13, 14].

Now, let's have a look at my more delicate methods...

METHOD 1

FACE STEAMING

Drainage from the outside (The preliminary stage)

The following method described in this section can be used to reduce an eye swelling. This is an advanced method of warm compresses. Warm compresses are limited as the towel or cloth continually becomes colder and the pressing action on the chalazion can irritate the tissue. A face steamer as shown in Figure 2 [11] is the best way to create a consistent high heat. The steam softens the skin, tissue and oils, allowing you to apply heat without touching the swelling, as in my case the lump would grow after each session when applying warm compresses.

One hour a day really softens the deepest oils and tissue of the chalazion. My chalazion actually began to move forward, from the inside to the outside surface of my eyelid, so that there was very little skin on the outside. The yellow colour was more prominent, but I felt this was progress at the time, as the chalazion was not growing in size anymore like it would when irritated by applying the warm compresses. Although it now looked worse in one way it felt like the stages of its life were being progressed. I could also now soften the lump much quicker.

After a few sessions on the face steamer all approximately half to one hour long, the chalazion began to drain from the outside. Over time a small dot or head began to appear during the face steaming sessions. This spot slowly released the oils after each session for around five minutes and then sealed up.

This method should mainly be used to soften the chalazion but it can also be used to drain from the outside surface. This should be taken carefully so that it is completed safely. I felt that over-steaming could open the head too much and could leave me in more trouble. I would recommend checking the condition of your skin on and around the swelling regularly so that the tissue is not over softened as the chalazion may burst if this process is pushed too far. Please be careful. I would recommend that the first time is perhaps only ten minutes long to be on the safe side. Different people will be at different stages, some with the lump very close to the outer skin, which will soften faster with steaming.

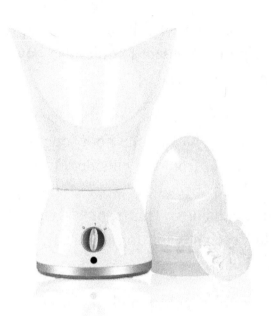

Fig. 2: A similar face steamer to one I used. Please find on Amazon.

Summary:

- Steam for around 1 hour at a time (Start with perhaps only 10 minutes in the first session). Check condition throughout the session every ten minutes or so that you will not over soften.

- Try to soften the oils deep within the chalazion over time, do not rush it.
- Bring the lump to the outer surface slowly over several sessions until a head is created in the form of a little yellow dot.
- If you wish to drain using this method gently push the swelling after steaming to drain the oils slowly, making sure not to irritate the chalazion as it may swell up further after the session. (This did not happen to me but the experience with warm compresses has shown this may happen).

Although I was progressing with this method I realised that drainage from the outside wasn't solving the real problem, the cause of the blockage. At this stage you would have been deeply softening the oils multiple times. I would then recommend moving to Method 2.

METHOD 2

CRYING NATURES WAY

Drainage from the inside (The final stage)

The following method described can be used to reduce an eye swelling to nothing with a natural and pain free technique.

I obviously cannot guarantee that it can work for everyone, as there are many stages and variations. Typically people on the forums say they are suffering up to 2 years before having to resort to surgery as this is what the doctors suggest. Two years is a very long time to carry a swollen lump around for, I had mine for a few months and really hated it.

Simply put Method 2 allows the blocked duck to open and the contained oils to be released. As the oils are flowing out this also helps to push through the cause of the blockage.

Richard James Clapham P.hD. Bioinspired Robotics
© 2016 copyright

To do this the best method is to rub a very freshly cut onion slice on to your chalazion. Within a few seconds your eye will begin to water and you will see the oils sitting / collecting on the inside of your eye. Some people may be more sensitive to the onion juice and vapours and their eye may water before the onion slice is close to their eye. If you are struggling just hold it as close as you can for as long as you can. Maybe if you start to see it working you get braver and will be more up to the rub as it is definitely recommended to massage the swelling with the onion to help significantly release a greater flow of oils and hopefully get that blockage removed completely.

By using both methods together the chalazion is sure to reduce in size and hopefully clear the cause of the blocked eye duct. Once your chalazion has been regularly softened Method 2 will work the most effective. You could try Method 2 first as it is the quickest and easiest way to get started but be very careful as Method 1 should ideally be undertaken first as this allows you to soften the whole chalazion thoroughly so that it will not be irritated during the process. Don't worry if it doesn't work straight away, it most probably will take a combination of the two as it did for me.

Once the chalazion was on the back ropes I would wake up in the morning to find that little yellow crust stuff on my eyelashes that you got when you were a kid. This was the swelling reducing in size overnight and was great to see in the morning. Finding this natural method to release the blockage was great for me. Rubbing the onion onto the eyelid stings of course but will make you cry so much which is what we need.

After the technique was proven to work I did get lazy leaving it maybe a month / a couple of weeks / maybe even two months and it always worked just as well as at the beginning. Even when the lump seemed to be hard and I was worried it wasn't fluid any longer. Currently I am left with just a little bit of dry skin which can barely be seen. I certainly don't get everyone pointing and going "your eye" and pulling a face of disgust.

This is by far the best method I found and wish I knew this at the start. Hopefully you haven't suffered too long with yours up till this point. I hope you have success too. I'm sure you will ☺

Richard James Clapham P.hD. Bioinspired Robotics
© 2016 copyright

Summary:

- Try to smoothly and gently massage the freshly cut onion segment into the swelling.
- You will see the oils release into the eye.
- 5 minutes after a successful try the swelling will be noticeably smaller.
- If unsuccessful go back to Method 1 until the chalazion has been softened more regularly and thoroughly so that the deepest parts are softened.
- You don't need to remove all the oils from the swelling in one go. Be patient, if you release a little of the oil you know that Method 2 will now work and you can successfully drain the chalazion.

CONCLUSION

This book provided a short and concise overview of chalazions, identifying the differences, describing the causes and introducing two successful treatments for draining a chalazion, by allowing the fluid to drain the natural way by opening the blocked gland. This method is by far a greater option then undergoing surgery. The two methods given should be ideally used in combination. Whereby the oils, tissue and skin are thoroughly and deeply softened multiple times, this will allow all of the swelling to drain effortlessly and fully once applying Method 2. Method 2 will drain the chalazion internally and naturally filling the eye with the contained fluid through the naturally processes of crying.

It was certainly a hassle once the chalazion appeared. I believe that it was caused by rubbing my nose after using a hay fever spray then touching my eyes. I spent many hours researching what it was and how I should remove/ heal it, ending up with no answers to the problem. Research is part of my background so I enjoyed that part during the time I had the chalazion. Although it was starting to affect my vision it was the going out in public I really hated. Unfortunately the lump was there for my VIVA exam as my research into the removal off the swelling could not be started in time. I certainly could not put up with eye swelling but cutting my eyelid open was going to be the last approach I would take. I vaguely remember having attempted piercing the chalazion but after reading this can cause infection and I felt this could really just increase the size and painfulness, I decided not to do so. I didn't feel comfortable with the thought of a doctor cutting my eyelid and then cutting the tissue away. My sister had a chalazion a few years ago and she was unable to reduce the size during the months she had it till it made her eye look wonky but we never told her that. She had to undergo surgery. Afterwards she said it hurt and was uncomfortable and her eye was really swollen. Just watching the procedure on YouTube was enough to motivate me to achieve my goal.

It has been a few months now and the chalazion looks like it won't be returning. I am now completely confident that even if I ever had a chalazion pop up again I could remove it no problem. I hope you have as much success as I did. All the best of luck! Go careful and cry your eyes out.

REFERENCES

[1] Understanding Styes -- the Basics:
http://www.webmd.com/eye-health/understanding-stye-basics

[2] Healthline Chalazion:
http://www.healthline.com/health/chalazion#Overview1

[3] Dambro MR (2006). Hordeolum (stye). In Griffith's 5-Minute Clinical Consult, p. 520. Philadelphia: Lippincott Williams and Wilkins.

[4] Neff AG, Carter CD (2009). Benign eyelid lesions. In M Yanoff, JS Duker, eds., Ophthalmology, 3rd ed., pp. 1422-1433. Edinburgh: Mosby.

[5] Trobe JD (2006). The red eye. Physician's Guide to Eye Care, 3rd ed., chap. 4, pp. 47-51. San Francisco: American Academy of Ophthalmology.

[6] Weinberg RS (2007). Diseases of the eyelid, conjunctiva, and anterior segment of the eye. In LR Barker et al., eds., Principles of Ambulatory Medicine, 7th ed., pp. 1816-1829. Philadelphia: Lippincott Williams and Wilkins.

[7] Wikipedia Chalazion:
https://en.wikipedia.org/wiki/Chalazion

[8] Wikipedia Cyst:
https://en.wikipedia.org/wiki/Cyst

[9] Wikipedia Stye:
https://en.wikipedia.org/wiki/Stye

[10] Removal of chalazion:
http://www.netdoctor.co.uk/procedures/surgical/a4671/removal-of-chalazion/

[11] Face Steamer Amazon USA:

http://www.amazon.com/gp/product/B0154YU2GI/ref=as_li_tl?i
e=UTF8&camp=1634&creative=19450&creativeASIN=B0154Y
U2GI&linkCode=as2&tag=homegrownwhea-21

[12] Chalazion and Hordeolum (Stye):
http://www.msdmanuals.com/en-gb/professional/eye-
disorders/eyelid-and-lacrimal-disorders/chalazion-and-
hordeolum-%28stye%29

[13] NHS: Chalazion – a lump on the eyelid:
http://www.guysandstthomas.nhs.uk/resources/patient-
information/eye/chalazion.pdf

[14] NHS: Treatment for a chalazion:
http://www.ouh.nhs.uk/patient-
guide/leaflets/files%5C090611chalazion.pdf

APPENDIX A – The Authors Background

Richard James Clapham holds a Ph.D. degree with the School of Computer Science and Electronic Engineering, University of Essex, Colchester, U.K.

His research interests include biological inspired robotics, mechanical engineering, marine robotics, fluid mechanics, embedded systems and intelligent control. He was the inventor of the robots *iSplash*-II and *iSplash*-MICRO the first robotic fish to outperform the swimming speed of real fish measured in BL/s.

Richard James Clapham is a Reviewer of the IEEE conferences ICRA and IROS. Is the author of four international conference papers, one journal paper and one book chapter.

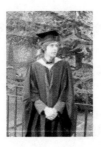

Richard James Clapham

Please help me by not replicating/ posting this
book or its content across the internet.

Thank You